EMERGENCY CHILDBIRTH: THE BABY IS COMING NOW!

A Helpful Guide When a Trained Attendant is Not There... or You Can't Make it to a Hospital or Other Facility!

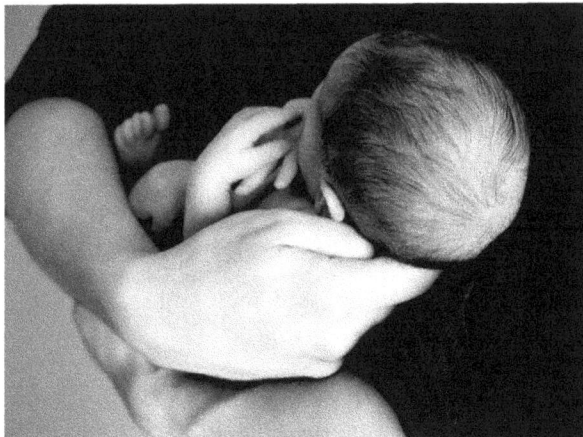

By
Victor M. Berman, MD
Salee Berman, CNM
with Marjie & James Hathaway, AAHCC

Dedicated to our grandson Roger Berman, who had an unintended home birth.

The Bradley Method® and American Academy of Husband-Coached Childbirth® are registered Trademarks with the U.S. Patent Office.

AAHCC

Academy Publications, Box 5224, Sherman Oaks, CA 91413

ISBN:0-931560-08-8

©2020 AAHCC

ISBN 978-0-931560-08-8

90000

9 780931 560088

© 2020 AAHCC

EMERGENCY CHILDBIRTH (QUICK GUIDE)

The following suggestions were edited from *Emergency Childbirth*, a joint publication of the U.S. Department of Defense, Office of Civil Defense, the U.S. Department of Health, Education and Welfare and the American Medical Association. Although it was first written for families who might have to take refuge in fallout shelters, the physiologic process of birth hasn't changed, so the same advice could be applied to most emergency births: in the car on the way to the hospital, snowstorms, earthquakes, floods, or any situation that would leave you on your own without medical assistance.

WHAT TO DO

1. Let nature be your best helper. Childbirth is a very natural act.
2. At the first signs of labor, assign the best-qualified person to remain with the mother.
   (Editor's note: a trained husband may be the best qualified.)
3. Be calm; reassure the mother.
4. Place mother and attendant in the most protected place.
5. Have hands as clean as possible.
6. Keep hands away from birth canal.
7. See that the baby breathes well.
8. Place the baby face down across mother's abdomen.
9. Keep the baby warm. *(Editor's note: Dr. Bradley says immediate breastfeeding will help expel the placenta, lower the risk of excessive bleeding, provide warmth [if baby is skin-to-skin with mother] and provide essential immunities for the baby.)*
10. Wrap afterbirth/placenta with the baby.
11. Keep the baby with mother constantly.
12. Make mother as comfortable as possible.
13. Identify the baby.

WHAT NOT TO DO

1. DO NOT hurry.
2. DO NOT pull on the baby; let the baby be born naturally.
3. DO NOT pull on the cord; let the placenta/afterbirth come naturally.
4. DO NOT tie and cut the cord until baby AND the placenta come naturally.
5. DO NOT give medication.

DO NOT HURRY - LET NATURE TAKE HER COURSE

Every expectant mother and the members of her family should do all they can to prepare for emergency births. They will need to know what to do and what to have ready. The Bradley Method® of Husband-Coached Childbirth trains instructors who advocate childbirth education. We do NOT encourage unattended births.

***

In addition to the above information, you may wish to read *Emergency Childbirth* by Gregory J. White, M.D.

Each family approaching the time of their child's birth should learn of the emergency medical facilities near their home. Are paramedics available? How do you get them? Which hospitals offer emergency care for mother AND baby? (Watch out - not all hospitals with an "Emergency Room" sign can deal with obstetrics.)

The front of this page is a Quick Guide...

Please continue to read the rest of the book
for more detailed information.

EMERGENCY CHILDBIRTH: THE BABY IS COMING NOW!
A Help Guide When a Trained Professional is Not There...
or You Can't Make it to a Hospital or Other Facility!

Victor M. Berman, M.D. Salee Berman, C.N.M.
with Marjie & James Hathaway, AAHCC

INTRODUCTION

Remember the stereotyped movie scene, with the woman screaming "The baby is coming." The midwife or country doctor comes and tells the frightened father to "go boil pots of water!" Nol one has ever figured out what the boiling water was for. The most likely explanation! was to keep the father out of the way. Today, we want the father to be there and be an active part of the birth team and we usually don't need tubs and tubs of boiling water. However, the problem remains, "What do I do now?"

This booklet outlines step-by-step what to do if "the baby comes" before the birth attendant or before starting to transport to the hospital and Mom says,
"I CAN'T MOOOVE! THE BABY IS COMING NOW"

This booklet is intended as a brief guide for the nonprofessional of how and what to do if you find that you are unable to get professional care in time to attend the mom who is giving birth. eg: Not able to transport to a hospital, happens in the car, or awaiting birth attendant.

This is not a guide for unattended midwife. The American Academy of Husband-Coached Childbirth, AAHCC, The Bradley Method®) and Victor Berman, MD and Salee Berman, CNM neither endorse nor support home birth that is not attended by trained professionals.

CONDITIONS REQUIRING IMMEDIATE HOSPITALIZATION-CALL 911

Childbirth is usually normal and the majority of women can do perfectly well in an emergency or unable to get to a medical facility without any help at all. However, some conditions can arise where professional assistance can make the difference between life and death. In this booklet, we will mention several conditions which call for immediate hospitalization. These will be emphasized by **(BOLD TYPE PRINT *)** which means " **CALL-911**, transport to the hospital immediately." By following this advice, lives will be saved. The care giver should discuss warning signs or problems that are occurring during the pregnancy. If certain conditions are present, home birth should not be attempted because of the serious complications that could occur. If you have been cautioned of problems, please arrange for emergency hospitalization in advance, including emergency transportation if mom finds herself at home alone when labor begins.

PREMATURE BIRTH*

Premature birth is more than three weeks before the estimated due date. Premature babies are prone to life threatening complications. Emergency life support systems and expert professional care should be immediately available.

TWINS*

The same thing applies here. Multi-birth may predispose a pregnancy to all kinds of problems and double the complications.

ABNORMAL PRESENTATION*

Breech, Transverse Lie, Face.

MOTHERS WITH MEDICAL COMPLICATIONS*

Diabetes, Essential Hypertension or High Blood Pressure, Bleeding During Pregnancy, Heart or Lung Disease, Bleeding Tendencies, Epilepsy, Any other serious medical condition requiring medication or ongoing medical care.

EARLY LABOR (Phase 1: Prodromal (pre) and early labor)

Beginning of contractions, softening, thinning and dilation of the cervix. Baby's head begins to fit into mothers' pelvis.

FIRST SIGNS

All of the following may or may not occur:

Bloody show (not heavy bleeding)

Contractions

Diarrhea Feeling of euphoria or apprehension

Frequent urge to urinate

Mucous discharge

Periodic low back pain

Ruptured membranes, (breaking of the bag of waters).

NORMAL LABOR (Phase 2: Active labor)

Before we consider how to deal with an emergency birth, a basic understanding of the process of labor is necessary.

Classically labor is divided into three stages:

First Stage   (1): From onset of labor to complete dilation.

Second Stage (2): Complete dilation to delivery of baby.

Third Stage   (3): Delivery of placenta.

(We have found it useful to divide First Stage (1) into three phases because women have different behaviors and needs at these times.)

Emergency Childbirth: The Baby is Coming Now! ©2020 AAHCC

Phase 1: Prodromal (pre) and early labor
Phase 2: Active labor
Phase 3: Transition

Any of these may be early signs of the onset of labor. Contractions may be so mild at first that Mom may hardly notice them. They may feel like light menstrual type cramps or may be strong right from the beginning. They could be as far apart as minutes, hours, or days. They could start off closer than five minutes. The word, "contraction," refers to the tightening of the uterine muscle and can be felt by placing a hand at the upper portion of the abdomen. Don't be afraid to press firmly (with care). Mom will tell you if you are pressing too hard. The uterus will feel firm during the contraction. When the contraction subsides the uterus gradually becomes soft. To get an idea of what we are talking about, press on your own biceps muscle and compare when it is tense and when it is relaxed.

TIMING THE CONTRACTIONS

Early uterine contractions usually last 20-40 seconds. Simultaneously, mom may feel some mild pain or cramping but as mentioned before, she may not feel much in early labor. When timing contractions, we are interested in **two things**, **how long** they last (**duration**) and **how often** they occur (**frequency**). If it is not too uncomfortable to the mother, you can time contractions by placing your hand on the upper abdomen and measuring the time from the first tightening until relaxation. Also note the time it occurs. Measure the frequency from the beginning of one contraction to the beginning of the next. If the laboring woman finds that this is uncomfortable, you can ask her to tell you when they start and end and time them in the same way. Doing this for about twenty minutes at a time will give you a good idea of frequency and duration. Keeping track of this on paper will help you to be able to report to your attendant. In early labor, contractions may last only a short time and may be as far apart as fifteen minutes or more. They are relatively mild to moderate in strength and usually not very painful. Labor averages 15-17 hours.

MUCOUS DISCHARGE

Mucus is a gooey, gelatinous substance that can vary from almost liquid to almost solid. It may be stained dark brown like old blood or pinky red. It may be clear, opaque or yellowish and have virtually no odor. A foul smell could be a sign of infection. **IF THERE IS A DEFINITE FOUL ODOR, HOSPITAL EVALUATION IS NECESSARY IMMEDIATELY. IN THIS CASE, ANTIBIOTIC THERAPY MAY BE LIFE SAVING FOR BABY, MOTHER OR BOTH***

MUCOUS PLUG

Many books mention the magical mucous plug that should be included in early signs of labor. We have found that it has no real significance. It may be present and it may not. If you see it, it closely resembles a mucous discharge or piece of crayon.

Emergency Childbirth: The Baby is Coming Now! ©2020 AAHCC

It has no relationship to whether labor is fast or slow, healthy or not. We suggest you forget it.

BLEEDING

A small amount of bleeding is normal in labor. Bleeding may take several forms. **HEAVY BLEEDING*** is rare and can be life threatening.

FORMS OF BLEEDING

1. BLOODY DISCHARGE.

Pink-diluted with mucus or other fluids. Red-new blood, undiluted Brown to black old bleeding(s).

2. **HEAVY RED FLOWING BLOOD***

If this bleeding is painless, it may be due to placenta previa. Rarely, the placenta grows low enough in the uterus to obstruct the cervical opening, either completely or partially. This condition is life threatening to both baby and mother and requires immediate hospitalization for a cesarean operation.

3. **RED BLEEDING ACCOMPANIED BY A TENSE, TIGHT, ABDOMEN WITH SEVERE PAIN.***

This also requires immediate hospitalization. This rare type of bleeding could be due to placental abruption, partial or complete separation of the normally implanted placenta prior to the birth of the baby. The baby's and mother's lives could be saved by an emergency cesarean operation.

RUPTURE OF MEMBRANES (Bag of Waters)

Membranes may rupture anytime in labor. As mentioned before, this may be the first sign of labor or it may not take place until the baby is born. It may happen with a gush or appear as a gradual trickle. The amniotic fluid may be clear or be tinged pink from mild bleeding. The fluid constantly replenishes itself and will continue to come out until the birth. It may be difficult to distinguish leaking fluid from a watery mucous discharge or urine which may be normal in late pregnancy. If leaking persists for more than a few hours, it should be reported to your care giver so that they can test it chemically. Leaking fluid has the same significance as frankly ruptured membranes.

FOUL-SMELLING AMNIOTIC FLUID*

Normal amniotic fluid is clear and fresh smelling. It is odorless or resembles the odor of clean sea water. **FOUL SMELLING AMNIOTIC FLUID*** is a sign of infection and could be a life threatening condition for mother and baby. Immediate hospitalization is necessary.

Emergency Childbirth: The Baby is Coming Now! ©2020 AAHCC

BROWN, YELLOW- GREEN AMNIOTIC FLUID*

As mentioned above, normal amniotic fluid is clear, may be tinged with pink and may have flecks of vernix in it. If the fluid is brown or yellow-green stained. It could be a sign of fetal distress. It may also be thick and cloudy. This condition requires immediate professional evaluation. (Vernix is a white substance on the baby's skin to protect it in a water environment.)

PREMATURE RUPTURE OF MEMBRANES

This is a somewhat confusing term. It is defined as rupturing of the membranes before the onset of labor and does not refer to a premature baby. However, premature rupture of membranes may occur in "preterm" or 'premature' labor and can pose an extra threat to the well being of the baby which may already be compromised by the fact that it is "premature"

PROLONGED RUPTURE OF MEMBRANES*

This is defined as more than 24 hours of leaking fluid. Labor usually follows the rupture of the membranes within a few hours. If it doesn't, prolonged rupture may develop. After the membranes are ruptured, they can no longer serve their function of protecting the baby and the lining of the uterus from infection. The treatment of this condition is beyond the scope of this book and must be managed professionally. Many physicians feel that the baby should be delivered within 24 hours of rupture of membranes. If labor is not established before this time, they are likely to consider induction or stimulation of labor. A mother with this problem should be hospitalized for further evaluation and care. Although this condition will be managed by the attending physician, these are some of the principles of management.

1. Expectant waiting (waiting excitedly).
2. **NOTHING** in the vagina, including vaginal exams
3. Temperature monitored every four hours or more frequently if infection is suspected.
4. Observe for signs of infection, such as fever and foul-smelling fluid.
5. Possible antibiotic therapy
6. Induction of labor

PROLAPSED CORD*

A prolapsed cord is more apt to occur in a mal presentation such as a breech because there is too much space between the baby and the cervix. However, a prolapsed cord can occur in any presentation. Emergency transport to the hospital is paramount. While on the way to the hospital the mother should be in a knee-chest position, which usually helps to protect the cord from the pressure of the baby's head. The father or attendant should put his hand along the side the baby's head, next to the cord, deep in the vagina and keep the head from pressing on the cord. This is awkward, uncomfortable and embarrassing but could be life saving.

FIRST STAGE: Phase 2
ESTABLISHED LABOR -Active labor

We like to call this the active phase. Contractions increase in intensity and pressure/pain and become more frequent. The mucous discharge may become heavier. Some bloody discharge is normal due to small capillaries breaking as the cervix dilates but not heavy bleeding. During this phase, great changes are taking place. The cervix is both dilating and effacing or thinning out. The baby's head descends further into the pelvis.

Mom needs psychological and physical support. She may want to eat light, easy to digest food can be given. Fluids such as Jell-O, cranberry juice, apple juice diluted with water or even plain water and an occasional spoon of honey will help keep her energy levels up. She should be encouraged to drink at least one quart of fluid every four hours. Nausea is very common in labor and eating heavier foods could cause vomiting & discomfort.

She may want to move her bowels as the baby's head gets lower and presses on the bowel. Make certain you do not get this confused with an urge to push! If labor has become very strong and the mother suddenly says" I have to move my bowels, I can't wait" Get extra newspapers or towels and have her go in the bed. It might be that she really has to move her bowels or it might be the baby. It's easier to clean up a mess in the bed than rescue a baby from the toilet!

Urinating should be encouraged frequently, at least once an hour. There is a danger of the bladder filling too full and interfering with the descent of the baby's head. If this should happen, the mother may not be able to urinate due to the unusual pressure. A full bladder increases pain and could interfere with effective pushing. If the problem becomes severe, mom may have to be catheterized in order to relieve the pressure. To help avoid the need to be catherized, Mom should place her hands on top of her pelvic bone, below the baby's head and attempt to lift the baby off her bladder while trying to urinate.

The most important factor is **PSYCHOLOGICAL SUPPORT**. She should be constantly reassured that all is going well and that labor is progressing normally. Remind her frequently, **"YOU CAN DO IT .. YOU ARE DOING IT."** Many women say in labor, "I'm not doing as well as that woman in the childbirth film. I don't think I can do this." She needs reassurance of how well she is doing. Remind her that most of the labor in the movie was edited out of the final film that she saw. Normal labor progresses at its own pace.

MUSIC may help her to relax, as may listening to her favorite poetry. Recorded sounds of nature are very relaxing to many women. Use whatever works.

PHYSICAL SUPPORT goes along with psychological support. Sitting in a warm tub has a wonderful relaxing effect as well as massage and soothing words. For many women, physical touch is almost hypnotic at this time. Lying in a very comfortable position with lots of pillows for support is helpful. Vary the resting by taking short brisk walks. If she has a contraction while walking, she can relax by draping herself over her husband by putting her arms around his neck and letting him completely support her. Help her to get into a more comfortable position. Suggest alternative positions. Help arrange pillows. Get cold compresses for her head. All of these things can be done by assistants. It is a practical way to involve friends and family to feel and be useful.

WHEN ITS TIME...

WHEN IS IT TIME TO GO TO THE HOSPITAL???
Hard to say... Many Factors! Check with your Birth Attendant.

WHEN IS IT TIME TO CALL THE BIRTH ATTENDANT?
Remember that a second or subsequent labor usually goes much faster than a first labor. If you are planning a hospital birth, discuss transportation to the hospital with your care giver. Find out when they want to be notified that you are in labor and when they want you to come to the hospital. Find out where to go once you get there. Many couples make practice runs to make sure they are familiar with the route and know how much time it will take.

If you have planned a home birth, you should have a clear understanding with your birth attendant. This should be included in your review of the birth plan. Find out when she wants to be notified, what she expects you to do, and when she is planning to come. How can you get in touch when you are in labor? Does she have a beeper? A portable telephone? After she is aware that you are in labor, she will keep in touch to see how things are progressing so she can make an educated judgement call when to come to your home. She will also want to reassure you and herself that labor is progressing well without any problems. **ANY UNUSUAL OR WORRISOME EVENT SUCH AS HEAVY BLEEDING, SEVERE PAIN, OR PROLONGED RUPTURE OF MEMBRANES NEEDS TO BE EVALUATED AND ALL COULD BE REASONS FOR HOSPITALIZATION.**

TRANSITION: Phase Three
Transition is the time between completion of dilation and the beginning of pushing. Sometimes this can be very long, particularly with first time labors. In a first labor, two to three hours is not unusual. In second or subsequent labors, transition is usually much shorter. Fifteen minutes to an hour is common and we have seen it as short as two or three contractions. As are all phases of labor, this phase is extremely variable from one woman to another. At this time tremendous emotional as well as physiological changes are happening. All attention must be focused on her. Hopefully, you have reached the hospital or your attendant is with you by now.

THIS COULD BE THE TIME WHEN MOM SAYS. "I CAN'T MOOVE. I HAVE TO PUSH!!!"

SECOND STAGE: IMMINENT BIRTH - WHAT DO I DO NOW?
At this point you have determined that it's too late to go to the hospital, or your birth attendant has not arrived.

First: Keep calm. Emergency, Fast, or Unexpected location births are usually healthy and normal. Your calmness will help to reassure mom. This reassurance will result in an efficient and cooperative birth.

Emergency Childbirth: The Baby is Coming Now! ©2020 AAHCC

Second: Give encouragement. Try and emphasize normality, such as "You can do it," "Everything is going well," "The baby will be here soon."

Third: While keeping calm and giving encouragement, be alert and always on the lookout for signs of problems.

Fourth: If there is enough time, collect the following:

Several clean towels

Wash cloths

Basin for placenta

Newspapers or underpads

Trash bags

Baby blankets and clothing

Surgical lubricant or Olive oil

Sharp scissors

Cord ties

Bulb or ear syringe

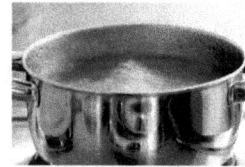

Small pot to boil water to sterilize scissors, cord ties and ear syringe.

AH HA! THAT'S WHAT THE BOILING WATER IS FOR!

HOW TO HELP A WOMAN GIVE BIRTH

Let us state in the beginning that the average woman with a healthy pregnancy will do well in labor and give birth unassisted. Ingrained fear is the greatest enemy. We will describe some ways you can help to make the process easier and warn you of a few problems which can occur and how to deal with them or when professional help can be life saving.

POSITIONS First & Second Stages

Get Mom in a comfortable position. The illustrations show several possibilities. We have found that the side-lying position with the coach helping to support the upper leg is usually easiest and at the same time more comfortable for most women, but everyone is different.

Suggest positions and try to find out what is best for her. Encourage her to relax.

If in a semi squatting position, get arms around both legs. If in a side-lying position, try to get an arm around the upper leg and pull back. Open your legs and make enough room for the baby to get through.

"Take several slow deep breaths---hold the next one--and push--not too hard. Imagine you are opening up the vagina. Hold your legs towards your chest and not too wide apart. " (this helps to prevent tearing)

The laboring woman must do this pulling and pushing herself. If you try to do it for her, she will instinctively move into the opposite direction and the purpose will be defeated. You can only encourage, suggest, and help her to get into a more comfortable position.

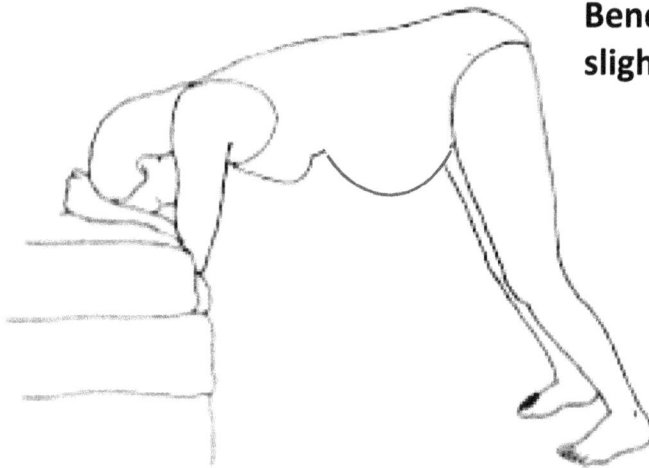

Bending over bed (bend knees slightly to relieve tension)

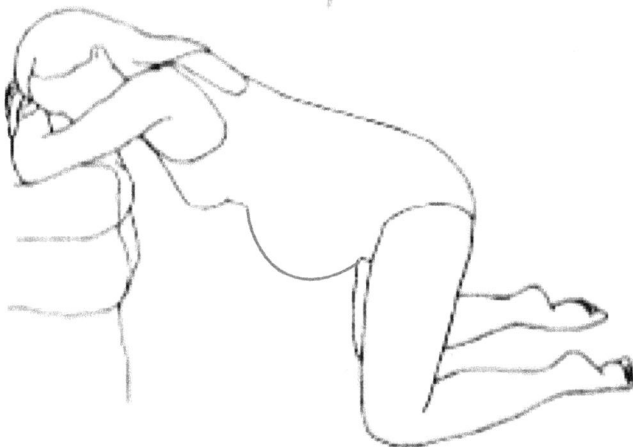

Kneeling against bed

Sitting in rocking chair

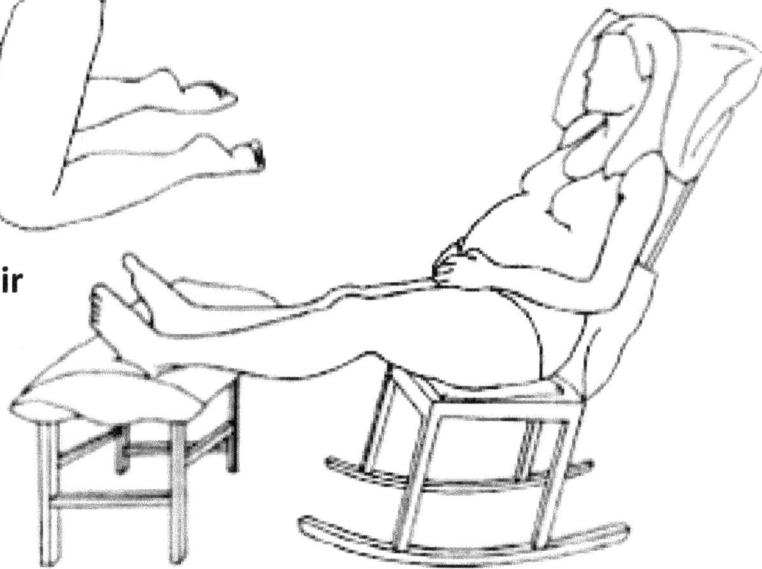

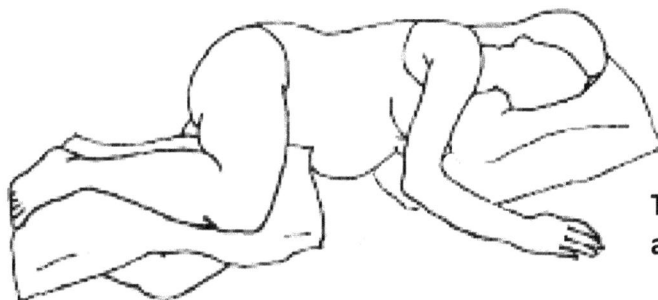

Total relaxation: pillows under head, arms, and abdomen, and between thighs

Side positions is most popular in First Stage

11

Semi-squatting during pushing

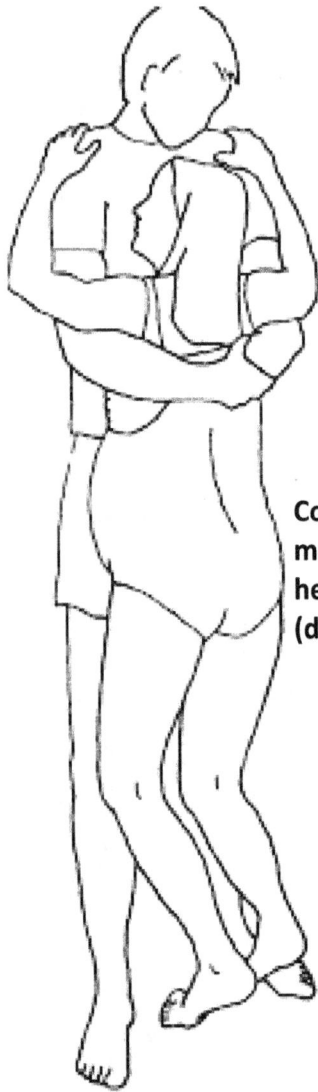

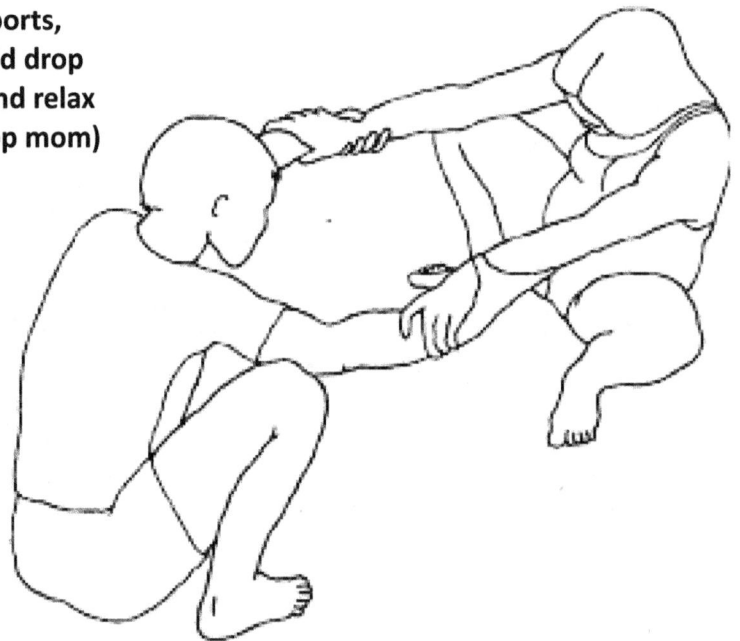

Coach supports,
mom should drop
her arms and relax
(do not drop mom)

Walking during a contraction,
supported by the Coach

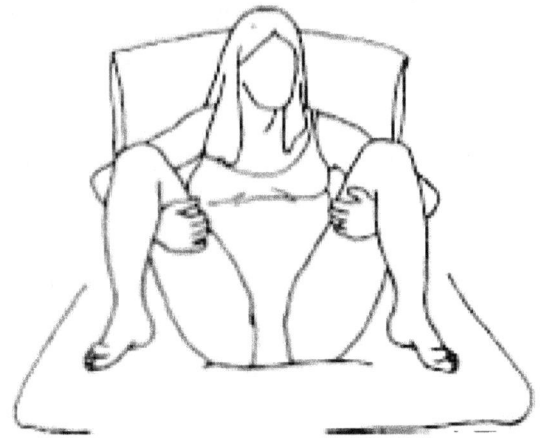

Squatting, with the Coach's support

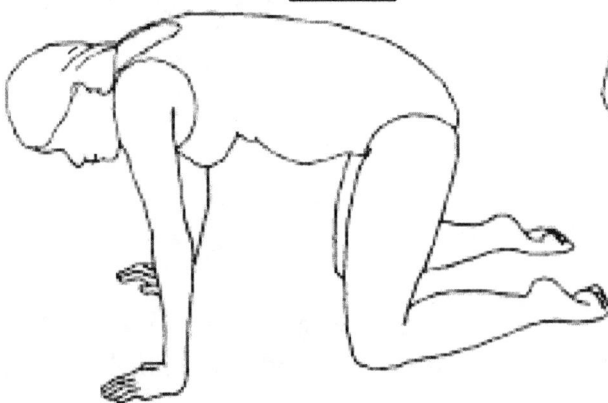

Pelvic rock: back straight and pelvis tucked in

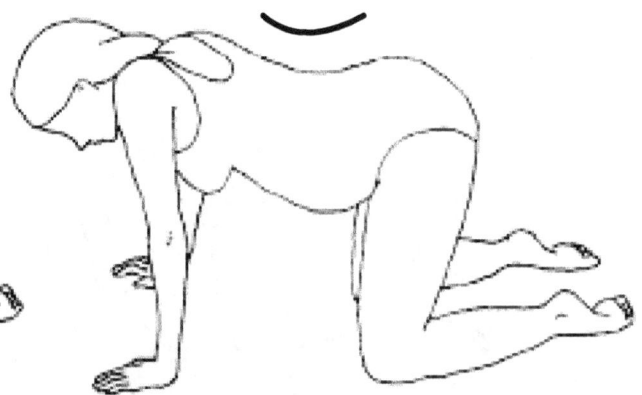

Pelvic rock: completely relaxed, abdomen hanging

PUSHING Second Stage

A frequent mistake is made by encouraging a woman in labor to push too early and too much. There are a few, very few, times when a woman should be encouraged to push hard and even fewer when she should be encouraged to push "as hard as she can." There are many dangers in pushing too hard too early. These include swelling of the cervix, swelling of the perineum, lacerations, discouragement, swelling of the bladder and not having enough strength left when she really has to push. Please don't exhort her to push any harder than she feels like, especially when she first starts to push. In fact, she should try not to push when she first feels the urge even though she wants to. When it is impossible not to push, encourage her to push just enough to help bear the contraction. Tell her to "save your strength for later." Pushing hard too early will only wear her out.

As the baby reaches the **vaginal opening**, you will be able to see the head. At first, just a bit with the height of the contraction, "a nickel's worth." After a few more pushes, "a quarter," and finally crowning, a whole silver dollar or more. Once again, we must remind you that this is so variable from one person to the next. In a second or subsequent birth this process may take only a few contractions. Another woman, especially if it is her first labor, may take several hours from the first glimpse of the head until birth.

As the **head crowns**, the whole perineum bulges. You may be able to see almost the entire outline of the baby's head bulging the perineum. The baby is almost ready to be born. Many women get discouraged at this point. Encourage her to put her fingers on the baby's head at the entrance to the vagina. Not only is this a thrilling once-in-a-lifetime feeling, but it drives home, in a practical way, the fact that the baby is almost here, that the labor process is almost over.

As the head pushes **against the perineum**, she may complain of a **TREMENDOUS BURNING SENSATION** from the skin stretching. This is a normal feeling. The head will soon be born and the burning sensation will be only a memory. Reassurance is all that is necessary. Frequently she will be in a state of altered consciousness at this phase. She may act as if she can't hear you but she does and is aware of everything that is going on. **NEVER UTTER A DISCOURAGING WORD. NOT EVEN BY GESTURE OR GRIMACE OR BODY LANGUAGE SHOULD ANYONE IN THE ROOM GIVE HER ANY NEGATIVE FEELING.** Constantly be encouraging. Say encouraging things. Think encouraging thoughts. Don't talk about anything but her and what is going on at the moment. This is not the time to talk about the news or what you did yesterday or what you are planning for tomorrow. Anything you say can and probably will be misinterpreted. At this point, she is the center of the universe and nothing matters but the successful birth of her baby. This is how it should be!

The baby is now **almost ready to emerge**. Now is the time, when with your help and her cooperation, you can work together to prevent or minimize tears or lacerations. There are several things you can do.

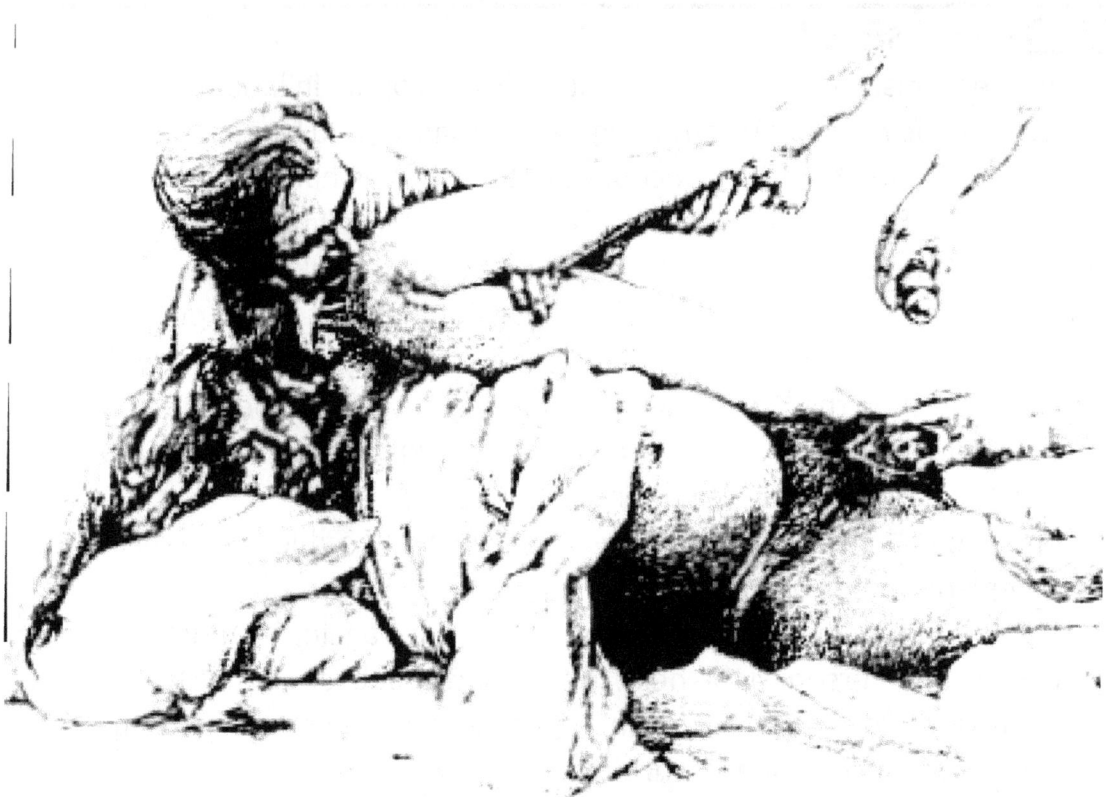

Push only as long and as hard as the pushing feels good & productive

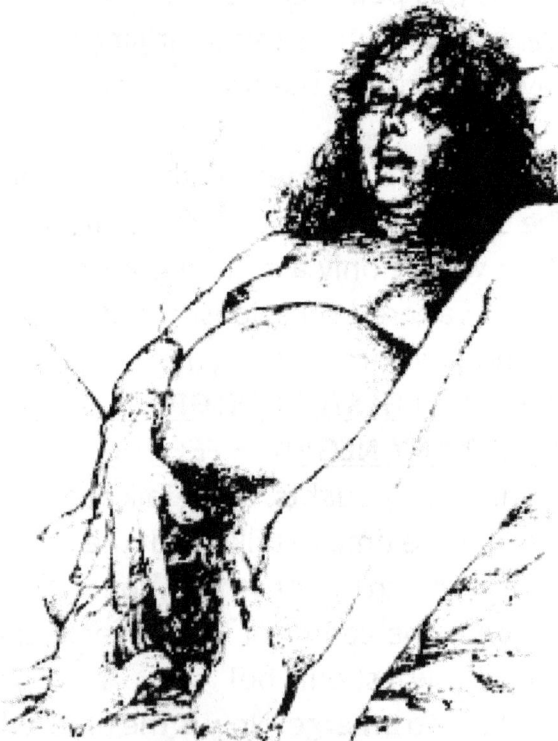

The unique feeling of touching the baby's head just before it is born.

HOT COMPRESSES

Ring out fresh wash cloths or towels in hot water and apply to the perineum just above the rectum. This helps to soften the perineum and prevent it from tearing. Explain what you are about to do before you do it. Most women like the feel of the hot compress. The compress should be hot but not hot enough to burn. Also use the hot towel to apply pressure to the perineum just above the rectum to help her to concentrate on the spot to focus pressure when pushing.

LUBRICATION

Use olive oil or other lubricant if available, not Vaseline. Pour a small amount of lubricant on top of the baby's head and into the vaginal opening. Go all around the bottom and sides but avoid the top. Not only does this help to prepare the tissue for stretching but also helps the baby to slide out with minimal injury to the mother.

The head is now about to be born. If possible try to ease the head out as gently as possible so as to avoid tearing of the perineum. Do not encourage strong pushing at this time! Tell her to push as little as possible and let the uterus do its own work. Allow the head to come out as gently as possible. **Explain to her:**

> "Listen to me carefully. The head is ready to be born now. Allow the contraction to do its own thing. You want the baby to come out as gently as possible. This will reduce the likelihood of tearing." "As the head comes out, **LET IT SLIDE OUT AS GENTLY AND SLOWLY AS POSSIBLE.**"

If the head seems to move out too quickly, try to gently hold it back and not push as hard. A frequent cause of perineal tears is too rapid expulsion of the head.

At this time, if the membranes are still around the baby's face, tear them away with your fingers to ensure that the baby can breathe when ready. This is rarely needed.

Support the head at this time with a warm, wet towel firmly held just above the mother's rectum, the same place you were pushing in when she was pushing the baby down a short while ago.

By doing this, you can also protect the head from contamination with feces because the pressure of the baby frequently causes mom to move her bowels. Allow the head to slide out with gentle support.

Emergency Childbirth: The Baby is Coming Now! ©2020 AAHCC

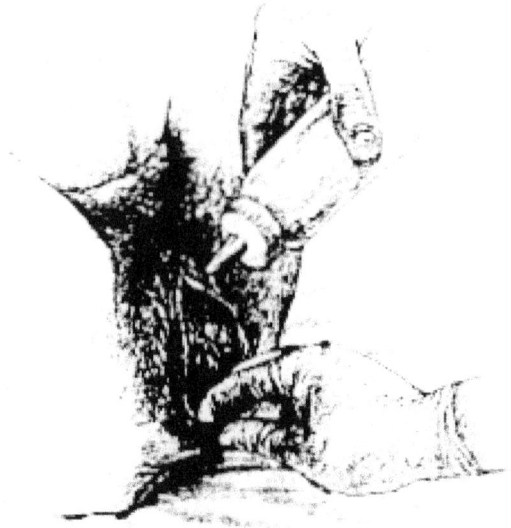

**Olive oil to
lubricate & soften tissue**

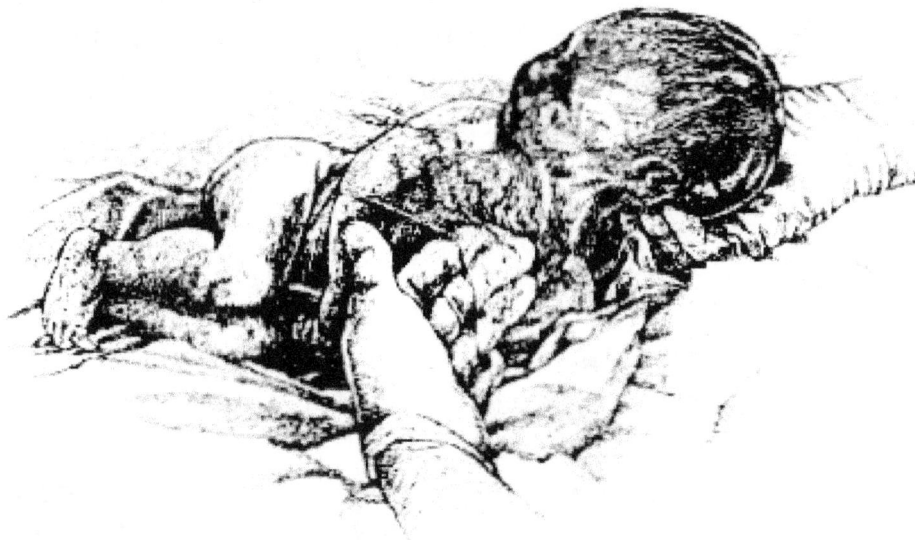

**Baby born "in the caul" (bag of waters membrane)
lift away so baby can breathe when ready.**

With the other hand, gently press downward on the top of the baby's head to prevent tearing. The head will usually come out facing down.

As soon as the head emerges, slide your fingers alongside the neck to feel for a loop of cord. We will describe how to deal with a cord around the neck in the section below. With the next contraction, the head will rotate to the side After the head has rotated, you can help by GENTLY pushing the head down so as to help the anterior or upper shoulder to come out. After the first shoulder comes out gently raise the baby so that the posterior or lower shoulder can come out. Be ready to "catch" the baby at this point. It might take a few more contractions or the baby might "shoot out" as soon as the posterior shoulder comes out. If the mother is in bed in any of the usual positions, you cannot drop the baby but if she is in a position where mom's buttocks are over the side of the bed, it would be possible to drop the baby. Be careful! Babies are very wet & slippery!

As soon as the baby is born, check to see that it is breathing. A lusty cry is reassuring but the baby may be perfectly healthy and breathe normally without a cry. Check for color. A normal baby may be a bit bluish for a few seconds but it will turn pink as soon as it takes a few breaths.

IF THE BABY DOES NOT BREATHE RIGHT AWAY, DO THE FOLLOWING:
(if necessary to stimulate baby to breathe)

1. Hold baby with its face to the side or down... fluid can then drain out.
2. Wipe the mucus from the baby's nose and mouth with a soft cloth.
3. If you have a rubber bulb syringe, use it to remove excess mucus from the baby's nose and mouth. Remember, always squeeze the bulb syringe **BEFORE** putting it in the baby's mouth. It should be placed in the mouth to the side. Release the bulb to suction. Otherwise, you will push mucus into the lungs instead of removing it.
4. Gently but rapidly rub the baby's chest.
5. Gently but rapidly rub the baby's abdomen.
6. With finger tips, gently and rapidly pinch the skin of the abdomen.
7. Blow on the baby's abdomen and chest. Your cool breath on baby's wet skin causes a reflex to deep breathe.
8. Rub gently but firmly along the spine.
9. If all of the above fails, use mouth to mouth artificial respiration. This is a potentially dangerous procedure in a newborn. Support the head and neck. Gently extend the head slightly backwards. Hold the baby's nose closed, place your mouth over the baby's mouth and puff (not blow) gently in the baby's mouth. Use only the air in your mouth for small puffs every three seconds.
DO NOT OVER BREATHE FOR THE BABY!!!

Emergency Childbirth: The Baby is Coming Now! ©2020 AAHCC

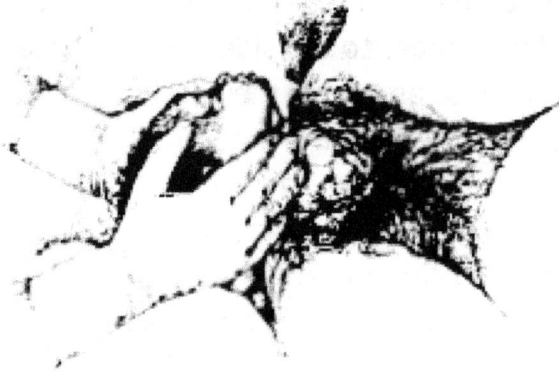

You can feel the vaginal pressure when the baby rotates to let the shoulders be born.

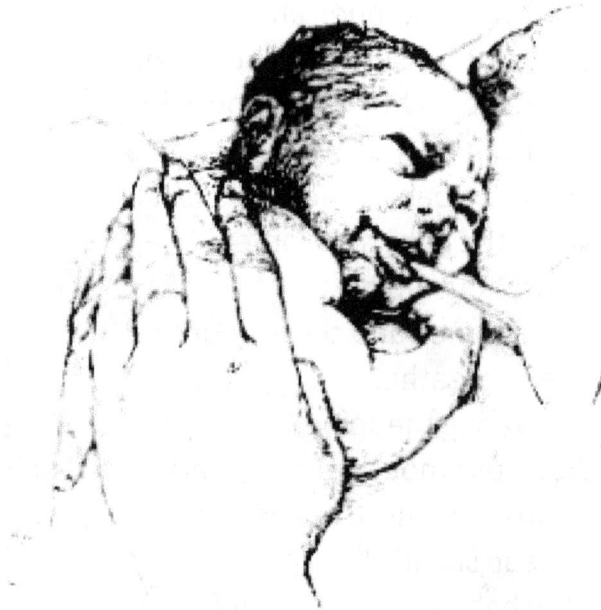

If necessary: To clear mucus; using a bulb syringe, suction the baby's nose and mouth with great care & gentleness.

UNUSUAL CONDITIONS

UMBILICAL CORD AROUND THE NECK (Head out of mom, baby's body still inside)

Occasionally, the umbilical cord will be wound around the neck. Slide your finger along the neck to feel for the cord. If it is there, try to reach in and lift a loop or loops of cord over the head. If it is too tight, try to pull gently on it so as to make enough room for the shoulders and body to slip through. The shoulders and body should deliver normally while you help to slide the cord over the body. Do not pull hard enough to tear it.

RUPTURE OF THE UMBILICAL CORD

This is extremely rare but it has happened so we will mention it here. If there is too much pressure on the cord as the baby comes out, it is possible for the cord to break in half. The broken ends will spurt blood. As frightening as this sounds, prompt action can prevent any damage. Grasp both ends of the cord from baby & placenta and squeeze them closed. Clamp or tie them as soon as is practical. If this is done quickly, there should be no problems.

SHOULDER DYSTOCIA- UNABLE TO DELIVER SHOULDERS*

Usually the anterior (top, facing up) shoulder follows the head in one or two contractions as described above. If it doesn't, encourage the mother to open up wide and push harder. Meanwhile check to see if the baby is breathing. If the baby is crying or definitely breathing, there is no rush to deliver the shoulders. If the baby is not breathing, turn the mother on her side. This will usually help to create enough room for the shoulders to come out. Encourage the mother to push **HARD. THIS IS ONE OF THE FEW TIMES WE NEED HER TO PUSH HARD.** Wait for two contractions and then attempt to help rotate the shoulders. There are two ways to do this. First attempt to push the posterior (lower) shoulder back with one hand while pushing the other shoulder down. If this doesn't work, attempt to rotate the entire body **IN THE DIRECTION THE HEAD IS FACING** by sliding one hand along the baby"s chest and the other along the baby's back. Another way of accomplishing the same thing is to slide one hand along the baby's back and catching the baby's armpit with your finger. In this manner, you can twist or spiral the baby so as to get the first shoulder under the mother's pubic bone. Once more, let us stress that this is an extremely unusual complication and the methods described should only be used while waiting for help to arrive, if the shoulder will not come out and the baby is not breathing.

IMMEDIATE CARE OF THE NEWBORN

Generally we try to keep the birth room quite warm. Even so, the baby has been used to the mother's body temperature. So, one of the first considerations is to keep the baby warm. Keep the baby skin to skin with the mother.

Emergency Childbirth: The Baby is Coming Now! ©2020 AAHCC

Put the baby to breast **immediately**, if the cord is long enough to reach. This will help produce contractions which help deliver the placenta and help to reduce maternal bleeding. If a baby nurses well, you can be reassured that the baby is in good condition. The baby's heart must be functioning well and breathing must be normal in order to nurse well.

CARE OF THE UMBILICAL CORD

Usually there is no rush to tie and cut the cord. We always try to wait until the cord stops pulsating and a resting state occurs (this could be 20 minutes or longer).

When the baby is first born, the umbilical cord will be thick and distended with blood & Wharton's jelly. You will be able to see it pulsate with the baby's heart beat. After a few minutes, it will change to a thinned out ribbon. The color will change from bluish to grey-white and you will no longer be able to see or feel pulsations.

The baby is no longer getting blood or oxygen from the cord and it may now be tied or clamped and cut. However, no harm will result from waiting many hours before doing this. You can wait for professional help as long as you wish. If you choose not to cut the cord, wrap the placenta in a blanket with the baby while waiting for your birth attendant.

There is no problem in clamping and tying the cord before or after the placenta is born. The way the cord is tied has nothing to do with the belly button. An "innie" or "outie" is determined by nature.

If you do decide to cut the cord, start at least 5 inches from the baby. It can be tied with light string, heavy cotton thread, surgical gauze, or the time-honored shoe lace. Wash and sterilize the material first by boiling it in water for five minutes.

Clamp or tie the cord securely with double knots five inches from the baby and then once more next to this for security. Then tie again, a third tie, about five inches further out from the baby and closer to the placenta. When you are certain that the ties are secure, cut with sterilized scissors, knife, or razor between them leaving the two ties on the baby's side. The purpose in the extra tie is to give extra security on the baby's side. This is the most important place because the baby would bleed from this site if it were not securely tied. The tie on the placenta side is to save blood in the cord for testing.

If the placenta is already born, do not discard but save for laboratory use. One reason for doing the cord early would be if the cord were too short for the mother to nurse and the placenta was slow in coming out. Another word about variability at this time, the length of the cord is different for every baby. It can be as short as 14 inches and as long as three feet.

Emergency Childbirth: The Baby is Coming Now! ©2020 AAHCC

DELIVERY (EXPULSION) OF THE PLACENTA

The average wait for delivery of the placenta is fifteen to twenty minutes but may be more or less. As long as there is no heavy bleeding the process should not be rushed. Observe the mother for signs that the placenta is ready to be born.

The signs of separation of the placenta are:
1. A sudden gush of blood.
2. A change in the shape of the uterus from oval to round.
3. Lengthening or pushing out of the umbilical cord.

After a few minutes, contractions will usually start again, similar to labor contractions but not as strong and painful. These contractions will help to separate the placenta from the uterus and help it to be born. Encourage the mother to push gently with the contractions.

Soon the placenta should come out, perhaps all at once or possibly a little at a time. This may take several contractions. In any case, **DO NOT PULL!** Have a large bowl ready to place the placenta in. After the placenta is born, feel the uterus just below the mother's belly button. If it is soft, massage it with your fingers. You will feel it get hard as you knead the muscle. Massage it until it is firm and round. This helps to reduce the amount of bleeding. Mom may complain that this is painful but if she is bleeding, **IT IS NECESSARY**! Explain to her why you are massaging the uterus. The baby should be nursing at this time.

When the baby nurses, it stimulates the mother's body to produce pitocin, the hormone that causes the uterus to contract. If the placenta has not yet come out, nursing helps to stimulate the contractions which help it to be born. As mentioned above, this might be a reason to tie and cut the cord before the birth of the placenta.

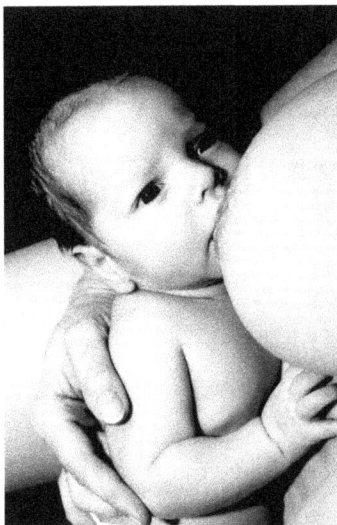

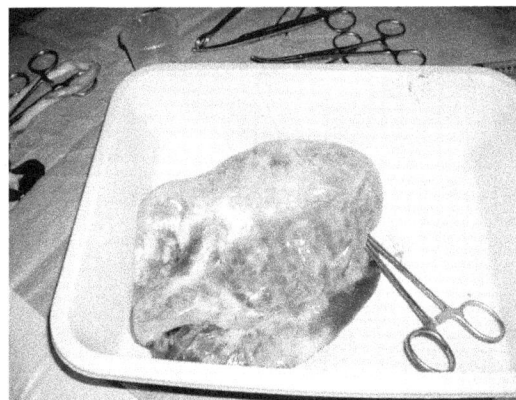

The Placenta looks like a blob that will be pushed out by contractions and gravity. It feels like delivering a bowl of Jell-O.

Emergency Childbirth: The Baby is Coming Now! ©2020 AAHCC

HEAVY BLEEDING WITHOUT THE BIRTH OF THE PLACENTA.*

If heavy bleeding continues and the placenta does not come out you must get the mother to the hospital immediately. Continue to massage the top of the uterus as described above until you can get help. **MOM MUST BE BREASTFEEDING...** helps contract and reduce the size of the uterus.

Sometimes the placenta comes out only partially and you may see membranes protruding from the vagina. If there is no unusual bleeding, you can wait for uterine contractions to push out the membranes. If they do not come out or, **IF HEAVY BLEEDING PERSISTS*** professional help is necessary.

Birth of the placenta is always accompanied by some bleeding but it should not be heavy. After the placenta is born, it should be saved so that the health professionals can examine it to be sure it is intact and nothing left inside mom.

POSTPARTUM HEMORRHAGE - HEAVY BLEEDING THAT CONTINUES AFTER THE BABY IS BORN*

After the placenta is delivered, you must still watch for heavy bleeding. Mother will continue to bleed and have contractions, the so called after birth contractions. These contractions help to constrict the blood vessels inside the uterus and nursing the baby helps to stimulate these contractions as well. **MOM MUST BE BREASTFEEDING...** helps contract and reduce the size of the uterus.

If the mother complains that the after birth contractions are very painful, explain to her that they are normal and are helping the uterus to contract If the uterus is not contracting well and bleeding is heavy, massage the fundus of the uterus as described above. If this, does not stop this **HEAVY BLEEDING*** transport the mother to the hospital. **MOM MUST BE BREASTFEEDING...** helps contract and reduce the size of the uterus.

LACERATIONS (cuts & tears)

Frequently there are small tears or lacerations of the vaginal opening. If these are very shallow, fit together easily and do not bleed, they will probably not need any treatment. Your birth attendant will evaluate any lacerations to see if they need suturing.

If there is a **LARGE LACERATION(cut) THAT CONTINUES TO BLEED HEAVILY***, she will have to be transported to the hospital.

EVALUATION OF HEAVY BLEEDING

We have mentioned **HEAVY BLEEDING** many times. Sometimes it is difficult to decide whether bleeding is really heavy. In general, try to estimate how the blood would fill an ordinary measuring cup if you consider all the blood, including that which is spilled on the sheets, or the floor. Do not include amniotic fluid or urine that may be mixed with the blood. If there is a full cup or eight ounces, **IT IS HEAVY BLEEDING**. If there are two full cups, it is **VERY HEAVY BLEEDING*** and the mother may begin to show signs of shock. These. include faintness, dizziness, fading vision, nausea, vomiting, fear, apprehension and a rapid pulse more than 120 beats per minute. The object is to get help **BEFORE** she shows signs of shock. Prompt action can minimize blood loss and prevent blood transfusions, shock or even death. While waiting for help to arrive, elevate the Mothers's buttocks and legs higher than her head. Try and keep the uterus firm by either massage or a very tight wrap around her abdomen.

SHAKING AFTER BIRTH

Shaking is normal after all the tension of giving birth. Sometimes she may be cold from sweating. Place a warm blanket over her & baby. Give her some **ORANGE JUICE**. The shaking should subside in a short while.

CHECK LIST FOR BABY:

BREATHING: Breathing should be unlabored, 30-40 breaths per minute. It is usually somewhat irregular. Normal newborn respiration frequently appears to stop for two or three seconds and then start again.

HEART: You will be able to see the pulsations in the baby's chest or feel them with a finger on the chest. 120-150 beats per minute are normal. Above or below that range, could indicate a serious problem and should be immediately evaluated professionally.

COLOR: An all over ruddy pink is healthy. Bluish palms of the hands and soles of the feet are all right but other blue elsewhere needs to be professionally observed, particularly around the mouth.

CORD: After it has been cut, make sure that there is no bleeding. If it continues to ooze, place another tie on it.

REFLEXES: The baby should have good muscle tone and have a good startle reflex. It should pull back when you pull on the extremities. It should also react when stroked.

BREAST FEEDING: Immediately after birth, the baby will begin to stick its tongue out and lick its lips. This is usually an indication that it is ready to start nursing.

Emergency Childbirth: The Baby is Coming Now! ©2020 AAHCC

Place the baby to mom's breast and it will latch on. Babies that have a good sucking reflex are usually healthy. A baby with problems or a sick baby will not nurse. The baby is getting the colostrum which is vital for its well being. It will nurse on and off for several hours and then be ready to go into a nice long sleep.

WARMTH: Keep the baby warm and dry to prevent chilling. Skin to skin with Mother is best. Place a large towel or receiving blanket over **both** mother and baby immediately after birth.

NEW BORN EXAM, EYE CARE AND SCREENING: Within two hours of the birth your health care provider should do a complete examination and assessment of the baby. They will follow through with eye care, newborn screening, immunizations and vitamin K.

CHECK LIST FOR MOTHER:

BLEEDING

Use the extra absorbent large size menstrual pads (not tampons), two at a time for the first 24 hours after birth. It is common to see a few blood clots. Soaking through a pad per hour after the first hour is considered **HEAVY BLEEDING*** and must be professionally evaluated. Normal bleeding will gradually slow in a few days. After about ten days, it is a mere trickle and usually stops by four weeks.

LACERATIONS (cuts/tears): Check the vaginal opening for lacerations. If they are small, fit together and stop bleeding after a short time, they might not need any treatment. If they continue to bleed, your professional care giver must evaluate them.

FUNDUS (Uterus) CONTRACTED: Check the fundus (Top or largest part of uterus) externally to see if it is firm. If it is soft, massage it as we previously described. You may push out a blood clot.

PULSE: A normal pulse range should be less than 120. It should slow down to about 80 beats per minute within a few days if everything is normal and there was no excessive bleeding.

BREASTFEEDING: Mom may feel exhausted as well as exhilarated after giving birth but she should be able to breast feed. However, she may need some help supporting the baby at the breast. There is absolutely no correlation between the size of Mom's breast and nipple and her ability to breast feed. Rarely, previous breast surgery may prevent successful breast feeding. In this case, still place the baby to breast as nuzzling is beneficial to both and will stimulate the release of hormones.

URINATING:

Shortly after birth, she should be able to urinate freely in normal amounts. There is concern if she continues to feel the urge to urinate and can only dribble out a few drops or none at all. The entire area is very swollen and sore from the birth. Warm compresses or warm water poured over the perineum should help to alleviate the problem. If she is still unable to urinate, your care giver will have to decide what needs to be done.

FLUIDS: Give orange juice, water and other fluids frequently. She will need to replenish all the fluids she has just lost. She should drink about three glasses per hour for the first few hours and then keep a pitcher by her side. Remind her to drink frequently and every time she nurses.

MOTHER UP TO URINATE FOR THE FIRST TIME

When the new mother gets up to urinate for the first time, which usually is one to one and a half hours after giving birth, there is a danger of fainting. Before getting up, the fundus should be massaged until it is a firm ball. This may cause a large blood clot to be expelled. The blood clot may be large enough to look like a small placenta. A clot, however, is dark like liver and has no cellular structure when you examine it. She should have double pads on and have a towel fitted like a large diaper. She must have support on both sides even if she protests that she feels strong enough to do it by herself. If she feels faint, have her sit down on the floor wherever she is. Even if she has never fainted in her whole life she could easily faint now. There is no danger in fainting but the floor can be extremely hard when it comes up and hits you! If she continues to faint or shows other signs of shock, she may have lost more blood than you estimated. If this is the case, she has to be evaluated for shock as described above under the heading; **HEAVY BLEEDING***

POST PARTUM EXAM FOR MOTHER

The new mother should be examined and evaluated by her professional care giver within a few hours after the birth. They should evaluate any vaginal lacerations to see if they need to be sutured. They will check blood pressure, pulse, temperature, respiration and will evaluate the firmness of the uterus and vaginal bleeding. In some cases they might feel it necessary to give the mother Pitocin to aid in keeping the uterus firm. The placenta will be checked to see if it is intact. If the mother is RH negative, they will make arrangements for Rhogam.

SOME GENERAL CONSIDERATIONS

WE DO NOT RECOMMEND HOME BIRTH THAT IS NOT ATTENDED BY TRAINED MEDICAL PROFESSIONALS.

However, if you are involved in an emergency, unexpected, natural disaster, etc., or isolated situation:

KEEP CALM

USE COMMON SENSE

HELP TO KEEP THE MOTHER CALM, RELAXED, COMFORTABLE, AND REASSURED.

REMEMBER THAT IF YOU DO NOTHING, BUT JUST ARE THERE FOR HER, APPROXIMATELY 90% OF ALL BIRTHS WILL BE NORMAL WITHOUT ANY ASSISTANCE.

IN SPITE OF THE ABOVE, BE ALERT FOR PROBLEMS.

CALL FOR HELP

Emergency Childbirth: The Baby is Coming Now! ©2020 AAHCC

PREGNANT???

Online

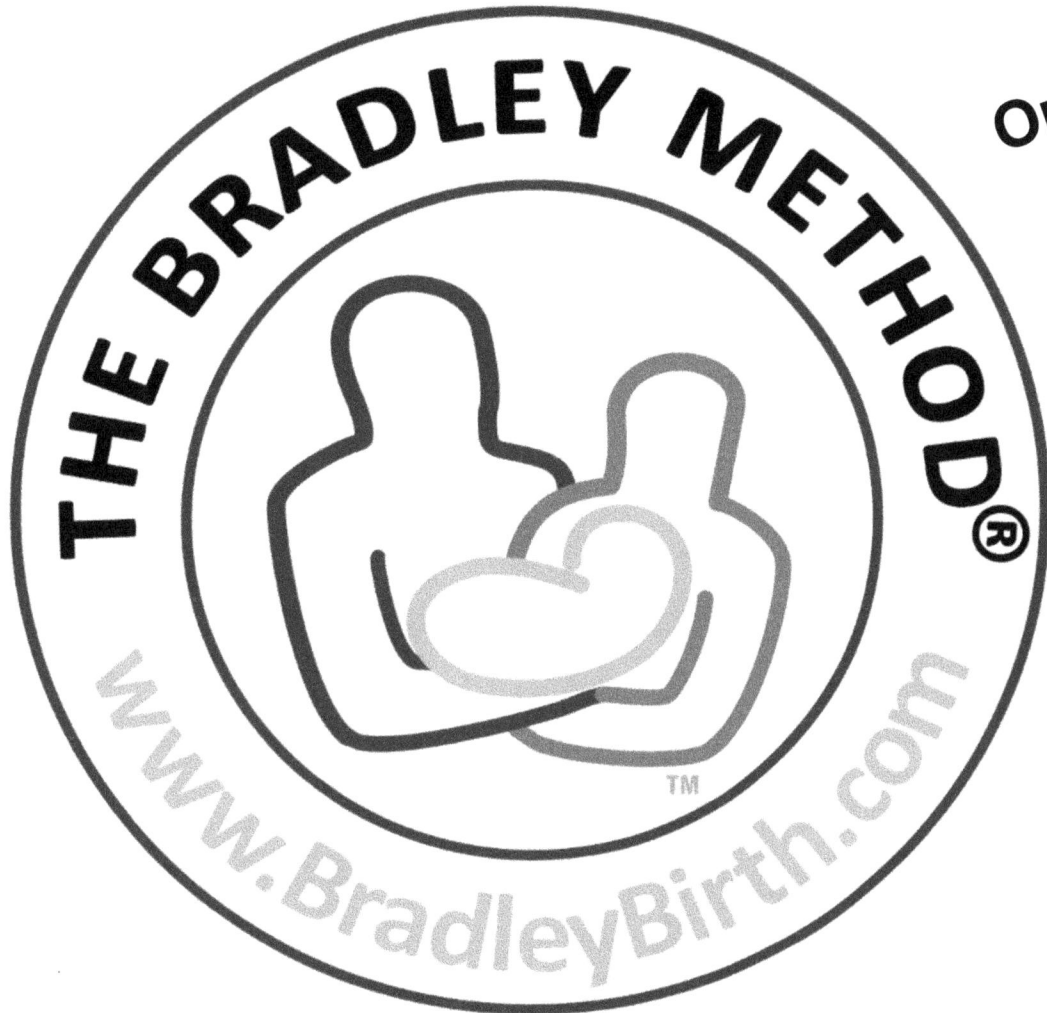

For Current Instructors & Access to our Online Hybrid Class Sessions go to:

www.BradleyBirth.com

Become a Bradley™ Teacher...
help us change the world!

Facebook: The Bradley Method® of Natural Childbirth